Fixing I

"A natural Hiatus Hernia Diet Treatment"

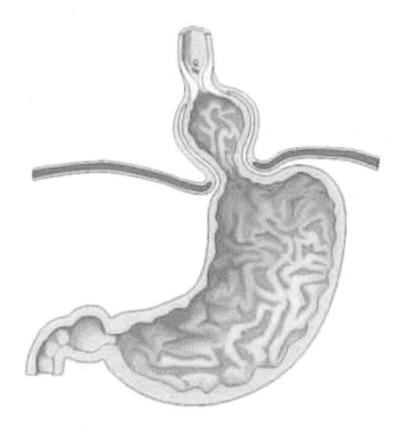

By Rudy S. Silva, Nutritionist

Hiatus Hernia: Diet For Recovering From Hiatus Hernia ©
2012, Updated 2014 Updated July 2018 by Rudy Silva Rudy S.
Silva

Printed updated 2018 in the United States of America

Table of Contents

TABLE OF CONTENTS 3

1: ALL ABOUT HIATAL HERNIA 5

2: HOW YOUR ESOPHAGUS AND STOMACH WORK............ 13

3: WHY YOU HAVE HIATUS HERNIA 19

4: WHERE TO START WHEN YOU HAVE HIATUS HERNIA.. 27

6: HOW TO TEST FOR AN ACID BODY 33

5: ELIMINATE AN ACID BODY-CREATE AN ALKALINE BODY
.... 39

7: BODY CYCLE THAT CAN FIX HIATUS HERNIA............... 49

8: FOOD YOU SHOULD EAT TO FIX HIATUS HERNIA 55

9: FIBER FOR YOUR HIATUS HERNIA RECOVERY.............. 65

10: WHAT TO DRINK TO STOP HIATUS HERNIA................. 71

11: SUPPLEMENTS THAT HELP ELIMINATE HIATUS HERNIA
.... 85

12: WHY VITAMIN D3 IS NECESSARY FOR HIATUS HERNIA
.... 95

13: EXERCISES NEEDED TO ELIMINATE HIATUS HERNIA
.... 103

14: ABOUT THE HIATUS HERNIA AUTHOR...................... 109

1: All About Hiatal Hernia

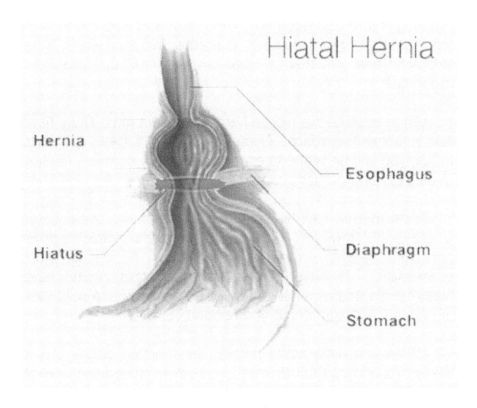

Hiatus Hernia

Hiatus Hernia, occurs when your stomach pushes back up into your esophagus or chest diaphragm. This occurs near the lower esophageal sphincter, LES. The opening or the aperture of the LES is called Hiatus. If the muscles and tissue in the LES become weak due to various strains and pressures, the LES becomes compromised. This allows the upper stomach to move into the esophagus and sets the stage for acid reflux.

Lower Esophageal Sphincter

The LES controls the passage of food from your esophagus into your stomach. It closes after you have eaten food so that your stomach contents will remain in your stomach, and so that it can't move back up into your esophagus.

When you have a hiatus hernia, you will most likely have acid reflux or heartburn. If you have frequent bouts with acid reflux, you will be prone to esophageal tissue damage, leading to an ulcer and perhaps cancer.

Hiatal hernia can be serious, but there are some cases where it not. However, if you have severe acid reflux, or other persistent health symptoms, then your hernia is more problematic.   However, there are many people who have hiatal hernia and experience few or no symptoms. A mild case of hernia is still something you need to correct.

When you have hiatal hernia, the function of the LES is weakened and can fail to keep stomach content from flowing back into your esophagus.   If your LES is strong then your lifestyle is causing your hiatus hernia.

Hiatus Hernia Categories

There are three categories of hiatal hernia – **reducible, incarcerated, and strangulated.**

In the **reducible** category**,** it is possible to push back the displaced stomach into its original position by gent pressure from outside of your body.

This gives you a chance to strengthen your esophagus and stomach muscles, using the information in this kindle book so that this hernia does not occur again.

In the **incarcerated** category, the out of place stomach cannot be pushed back manually, since it adheres to the surrounding tissue. The incarcerated hernia is not considered diseased or severe, but something that needs to be corrected. Using natural methods will help you eliminate this type of hernia.

In the **Strangulated** hernia, the stomach or esophagus tissues are tightly caught in the position they are in and their blood supply is cut off. This causes the tissue to eventually die. This is not typical, but when it does happen, surgery will be required.

Hiatus Hernia Symptoms or Conditions

The occurrence of Hiatus Hernia is quite common as you get older. Most likely, 50% of the people over 50 will get Hiatus Hernia, and many will not have symptoms. However, if you have pain behind your sternum, breastbone, around your nipple area and below, this could be because of Hiatus Hernia. The most common area to have pain is behind the breastbone.

If you have severe pain in the left chest, this could be mistaken for Angina, heart problems, or even acid reflux. Other symptoms for Hiatus Hernia are:

Ulcer: when you have an ulcer with Hiatus Hernia, you will feel a burning sensation along your esophagus area. This ulcer is created when you have acid reflux. The opening of the LES valve allows stomach acid to creep up your esophagus, causing an ulcer and giving you a burning sensation.

Hiccups: when your hiatus is large, hiccups will occur because of the irritation that occurs to the phrenic nerve.

Stooping: when you stoop or lie down, you will feel more pain.

Pain: the pain you feel can be like heartburn across different part of your chest and can be worst after you eat.

Bloating: you will feel full and have some bloating. Associated with this, you will have more bleaching and flatulence.

Vomiting: you may also experience vomiting. In some cases, you can have severe vomiting based on how severe your acid reflux or Hiatus Hernia condition is. Bloody vomit can be a sign of esophagus lining damage.

In addition, when there is an increased pressure in the stomach, caused by acid reflux, pregnancy, obesity, tight clothing, bending, straining, coughing, lifting excess weight, or overdoing exercising, hiatal hernia can occur.

Typically, there are no symptoms, when you have hiatal hernia. Since the LES is still functional, you may not have acid reflux. But, in some cases, you can have Hiatus Hernia and Acid Reflux and still have no symptoms.

Bleeding can occur in cases where an esophageal ulcer exists or where there is tissue degradation in the stomach tissue that is protruding.

Other Hiatus Hernia Symptoms

- Constipation
- Loss of hair

- Difficult breathing
- Difficulty Swallowing
- Dry mouth
- Bitter taste in the mouth
- Hoarseness in the morning or during the day
- Coughing at night
- Adrenal fatigue
- Heart attack like symptoms
- Food allergies
- Chest pain
- Abdominal pain
- Belching
- Regurgitation of stomach contents
- Unexpected weight loss
- Abdomen injury
- Age, over 50 with poor muscle tone
- Pregnancy

In cases, where there are large portions of the stomach that pushed through the esophagus hiatus, immediate surgery may be required.

Getting Rid Of Hiatus Hernia

Getting rid of Hiatus Hernia is not difficult, but it requires patience and persistence.

It requires following certain healthy practices. Knowing what these practices should be is the secret of eliminating your Hiatus Hernia. In this book, you will discover natural ways that you can recover your health. You will not only get rid of Hiatus Hernia, but you will also improve your overall health and experience a new energy and life.

Drugs

Using drugs for Hiatus Hernia can hamper your cure and prolong your recovery. In addition, expect some drug side effects. When you have Hiatus Hernia, you are not in the best of health. Using drugs will worsen your health condition since now your body has to deal with the toxicity of the drugs and your poor health.

There are many over-the-counter drugs that you can use to get temporary relief when your pain or burning feeling is related to acid reflux. You can use these drugs for temporary relief, but it is not recommended they be used long term.

Natural Methods to Health

Using natural methods to cure Hiatus Hernia is not just about using herbs and some nutritional supplements. But, it is based on eating the right foods at the right time. This will help you rebalance your body's chemist and to gain good nutrition, to eliminate hiatus hernia.

A natural cure will provide you relief in a relatively short time, but to get a full recovery will take some time. It took you some time to create Hiatus Hernia, so it will take some time to get your body back to normal. But, now is a good time to start living a different way.

The conditions that caused your Hiatus Hernia are related to the way you live. So, by changing the way you live to a healthier way, you can cure your Hiatus Hernia. Not only will you cure your Hiatus Hernia, but you be living a more natural way. This will improve your immune system and decrease the formation of many unpleasant and deadly diseases.

At the start of this program, you may have to be more diligent and consistent in eating good food, changing behavior, taking supplements, exercising, and detoxifying. Once you start to have some relief or start to see major health improvements, you can reduce the excess of this program and go into a maintenance mode.

In the following chapters, you will get information on how to eliminate Hiatus Hernia and acid reflux. Use and apply this information gradually and don't make radical changes in your daily habits. Gradually, add a few changes to your exercises, eating habits, and behavior each week. And over a months' time, you will start to see how good health practices benefited your health and reduce your hernia condition.

2: How Your Esophagus & Stomach Work

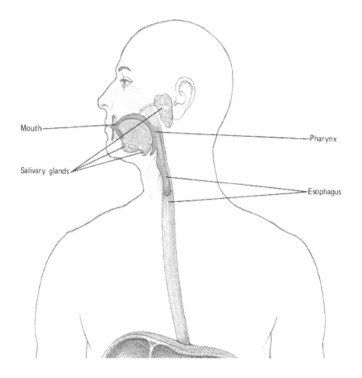

Esophagus

Once food is chewed, lubricated, and partially digested in your mouth, it becomes a bolus. To enter the esophagus, the bolus must pass the upper esophageal sphincter, which is a valve that is closed when no bolus is present.

The bolus then travels down the esophagus, by a contraction wave, to the valve at your stomach entrance, called lower esophageal sphincter, LES. This kind of wave is called peristalsis.

It takes nine seconds for a bolus to travel down your esophagus. If the bolus is liquid, it takes only 1 second. As food reaches your lower esophageal sphincter, the valve opens to let food into your stomach. The closing valve pressure of the LES is higher than the pressure inside your stomach. This condition does not let the bolus content and acid combination to flow back up your esophagus. It also prevents Hiatus Hernia from occurring.

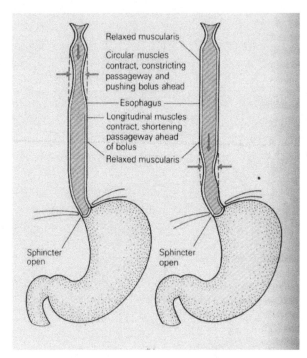

If for some reason, this valve opens and lets in digesting food, stomach acid, or parts of the stomach lining back into the esophagus, a burning sensation will be felt. This condition is referred to as acid reflux, heartburn, or GED, gastroesophageal disease. In the case where parts of the stomach move into the esophagus, this is called hiatus hernia.

Food Digestion

The digestion of your food starts when you are preparing your food. Cutting, dicing, mixing, pounding, or cooking, breaks down your food into small pieces, so you can chew and digest it easily.

Once in your mouth, saliva, which contain mucus, carbohydrate enzymes, fat enzymes, and bacteria start breaking down your food further.

Once you have chewed your food enough, it moves down your esophagus, within seconds, by quickly passing the upper and lower esophageal sphincter.

The lower esophageal sphincter must remain closed after your food moves into your stomach. If it does not, then you have a condition called acid reflux that can eventually lead to hiatus hernia.

How Your Stomach Works

To avoid having Hiatus Hernia or to stop Hiatus Hernia, you need to strengthen your LES value. To do this, you need to know how your stomach works and the things you need to avoid so that you don't interfere with the good function of your stomach.

Your stomach was made to be an acid chamber, so you need to keep it working as an acid chamber. As an acid chamber, it was designed to keep its pH 1.5 or less, and less is better.   When your stomach's pH moves above 3.0, your stomach automatically produces more acid to bring your pH down, below 3.0.

How does it move above a pH of 3.0? One way this occurs is when you take an acid reducer, acid blocker or drugstore Tums, or any other drugstore product designed to stop acid reflux or stomach pain.

Your stomach is happy and working like it should, when its pH is 3.0 or less because it can do its job, such as:

- Break protein into its individual amino acids

- Prepare vitamins and minerals to be absorbed in the intestines, such as vitamin B12, iron, calcium, magnesium, zinc, copper, and most B vitamins
- Destroy incoming bacteria and pathogens
- Reduce chances of coming down with stomach cancer
- Keep stomach content acidic, so when it goes into the duodenum, it triggers pancreas digestive juices
- Reduce chances of having allergies, skin disease, asthma, depression, lupus, grave's disease, osteoporosis, accelerated aging, and other conditions.
- Strengthens the LES value, so that the value remains strong and does not allow food or part of the stomach to push through and into the esophagus.

Using any type of drugstore remedies to get gas, pain, or acid reflux relief will weaken your stomach and LES valve.

In the following chapters, you will find the natural ways to follow, to maintain good levels of stomach acid. Good stomach acid is necessary for you to overcome Hiatus Hernia. Strong stomach acid is needed to influence and improve the absorption of nutrients that will give you better health.

Surgery

In some case, surgery may be required to correct Hiatus Hernia. Your doctor will be able to advise you in this area. When you have Hiatus Hernia, you may have to do a combination of drugs and a natural diet.

You will get the information you need, in this book, to follow a natural way to strengthen your digestive organs.

3: Why You Have Hiatus Hernia

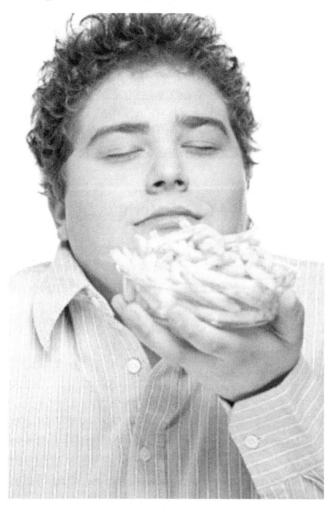

Why Do You Have Hiatus Hernia?

So the question is why do you have Hiatus Hernia? A lot of people might think that it is caused by an outside blow and by straining to lift a heavy object, but this is not the common cause. It has been found that 80% of the hiatus hernia occurs in adults over the age of forty-five.

Many people that have hiatus hernia don't have any symptoms. And, the symptoms that some people have can be related to acid reflux or heartburn.

A Hiatus Hernia can occur when the esophageal hiatus has been stretched and there is no actual tear in the tissue. This stretching can occur from weakness in the LES, or it can be that the hiatus is larger than normal, just from genetics. When these are the cases, then it is expected that the LES and its opening will stretch more as you age.

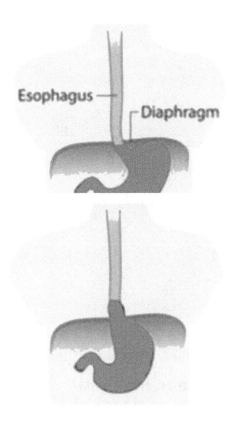

Esophagus

Diaphragm

Sliding hiatus hernia

Two types of Hiatus Hernia

There are two types of hiatus hernia that occur frequently. Here is what your esophagus and stomach should look like when you don't have hiatus hernia. Your LES valve and your stomach are slightly below your diaphragm.

When you do have hiatus that protrudes through your LES valve, this is called **Sliding Hiatus Hernia**.

This happens when part of the top stomach pushes into your esophagus. In this condition, the LES valve is weakened and you are more prone to having acid reflux.

This condition is not severe, but care must be taken so the condition does not worsen.

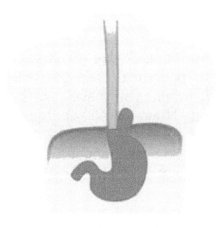

Paraesophageal hiatus hernia

The second hiatus hernia condition is called **Paraesophageal Hiatus Hernia**. This hernia condition is not typical. But, it is worse than a sliding hernia. When this hernia occurs, the esophagus and stomach remain in their normal position. But, when the stomach becomes congested or large, it can slide past the LES valve and settle along the outside of the esophagus and inside the diaphragm, the muscular area that lies between the chest and the lower abdomen.

There is a third type of hernia that occurs when you have both the sliding hiatus and the paraesophageal hiatus occurring at the same time.

Cause of Hiatus Hernia

The basic cause of hiatus hernia is having an unhealthy body, which is caused by having a poor living style. It comes from a poor diet, a toxic body, unhealthy thinking, and lack of exercises. It is caused by having an acid body, where you have an excess body acids that are causing your body to be imbalanced in digestion, absorption, and assimilation. This results in a weakness in organs and muscle tissue.

If you have a weakness in the LES or the LES is larger than normal, you will be more prone to hiatus hernia. In addition, if you have a poor lifestyle, forming hiatus hernia is more likely to occur.

When there is a weakness in the LES due to excess stretching, body acids, genetics, or poor diet, then the LES value can be further weakened, when you have excess coughing, reaching, bending, and lifting. All of these pressures work to weaken the LES further and over time the LES can open when it should not. When this happens, parts of the nearby stomach can move into the stretched LES opening.

When the LES opens it also causes acid reflux. Acid reflux and Hiatus Hernia go hand in hand, but they can also occur independently of each other. If you have Hiatus Hernia, then chances are that you probably have acid reflux.

More Reasons for Hiatus Hernia

There many other reasons why you might have Hiatus Hernia. People who are in their late middle age have a tendency to have a hiatus hernia, especially, if they have not followed a reasonably healthy diet.

Once you determine why you have it, you can avoid doing those things that have created your Hiatus Hernia. Here is a list of different reason why you might have this condition.

Smoking – if you smoke, you are nutritionally deficient and are more likely to have a hiatus hernia. Smoking uses up your alkaline minerals and your stores of anti-oxidants in an effort to eliminate the thousands of free radicals that you inhale.

With smoking, you end up with is a weakened body and especially a weaken esophagus and stomach area. With a weaken LES area, any deep coughing can create a Hiatus Hernia condition.

Constipation – many people suffer from constipation. You may have one bowel moment a day and still, suffer from constipation. If you sit in the bathroom for more than 4 to 5 minutes and you strain and push to have a bowel movement, you have constipation. When you strain, you are putting pressure all along the stomach wall and in the area of your abdomen.

Weak LES valve – with a weak LES, you can push a bit of your upper stomach in and out of the LES valve as you strain to have a bowel movement.

Overweight – when you are overweight, your stomach is enlarged, stomach acid is diminished, and the LES valve is weaker than normal. Most overweight people are prone to Hiatus Hernia.

Pregnancy – When you are pregnant, the pressures on your internal organs increase. The stomach area and the LES valve get distorted, which makes pregnant women more prone to Hiatus Hernia.

Excess Eating – when you over eat, your stomach will enlarge and move upward. If you have a weak LES or your valve is stretched out of shape, you will end up with Hiatus Hernia.

Allergies - food allergies can make your poor eating habits worse and add to the causes of a hernia.

Tight Clothes – anything that puts pressure on your stomach area can weaken that area. Wearing tight clothes or wearing a corset is not a good idea for good stomach health.

Bending – Here again, as you bend or squat, you increase the pressure in your abdomen. Over the years, this can create Hiatus Hernia. If you have poor posture when you sit or stand, this can affect the strength of your LES valve.

Belching – that occurs when you eat a mixture of too many foods or as a result of constipation or acid reflux, can produce Hiatus Hernia.

Exercise – lack of exercise is a health hazard. When you lack exercise, your metabolism slows down, your cells reduce their action, and your elimination channels reduce their activity. This is the best way to create an acid body and set yourself up for disease and Hiatus Hernia.

Acid Body – having an acid body is the worst condition you can have if you want to be healthy. You cannot have an acid body and expect to cure any type of illness you have, including hiatus hernia. An acid body makes you prone to all types of diseases and poor health conditions. To get rid of your hiatus hernia, you need to strive for an alkaline body.

Diet – eating good healthy food is necessary to maintain excellent health. A diet covers everything you put into your mouth, whether it is food or drink. Eating nutritious food will make your LES stronger and keep it close when it needs to be closed. This subject is covered in the next chapters.

Stress – Stress has a strong connection to the digestion of your food. When you have stress, the amount of stomach acid you have may be less or more causing poor digestion of your food.

Stress can cause you to overeat, eat junk food, and stop you from having healthy habits. Look for ways to reduce stress as this will be an important part of getting rid of your hiatus.

Stomach Injuries – any injuries or surgeries that affect the stomach or esophagus will have a weakening effect on your stomach function.

Smoking – smoking uses up the minerals you need to keep your body alkaline. It increases stomach acid inflammation and decreases muscle reflexes in the abdomen area.

Lifestyle Changes

Here are some lifestyle changes to consider. When making any changes ease into them. Make one or two changes then wait a few days to make another two. You want the changes to become part of your behavior.

- Instead of eating 3 large meals a day, try eating smaller meals throughout the day.
- Eat your last meal at least 3 to 4 hours prior to sleeping.
- If overweight, following the suggestions in this book will help you lose weight
- Eliminate or minimize drinking alcohol
- When sleeping, keep your head slightly elevated to prevent acid reflux.
- After a meal take a walk and do not bend or lie down.

- During a bowel movement, do not push or strain. Using plenty of fiber, using green drinks, and fruit smoothies will make movement easier.
- Wear loose clothes to prevent pressure in the stomach area.

4: Where To Start When You Have Hiatus Hernia

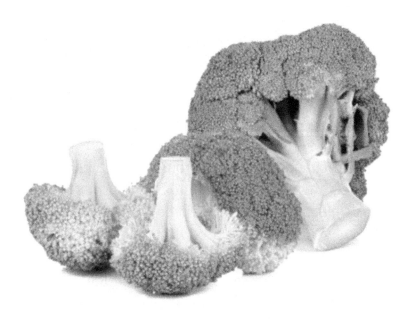

When you have a weakness in your LES, which is causing Hiatus Hernia and or acid reflux, then you need to strengthen and repair your esophagus, LES valve, and your stomach lining. You have to improve your digestion, make your body more alkaline, and eat the right kinds of food.

How do you do all of this without feeling overwhelmed and giving up before you start? First, you need to be dedicated and want to eliminate your Hiatus Hernia. If you don't concentrate on eliminating your hernia, it can get worse and lead to other more devastating diseases.

You can help your body produce a Hiatus Hernia cure. By knowing some powerful natural and nutritional ideas, you can make changes in your health that will eliminate Hiatus Hernia. Here is where you need to start.

1. pH Testing – the first thing you should do is test your saliva with a strip of pH paper. This will give you a pH baseline. As you go through the suggestions in this book, you can measure your saliva to see if your body is becoming more alkaline.

2. Acid Body – in the following chapters you will discover how to change your body from acid to alkaline. When you do this, you will start to see an improvement in your hiatus hernia condition. When you have acid reflux, your overall acid condition comes into play. By reducing your body's acid and moving it to a more alkaline condition, you improve your immune system and your body can fight your hiatus hernia condition more effectively.

3. Body Cycles – in the chapters that follow, you will find out how your body goes through certain cycles. By tuning into these cycles and providing your body with what it needs, during these cycles, you will create powerful steps to curing your Hiatus Hernia.

4. Next, you need to know what foods to eat and which foods not to eat. The foods you need to eat are 20% acid foods and 80% alkaline foods. The condition you want to achieve is an alkaline body. It is this type of body that works to prevent disease of all types.

5. You want to increase the amount of fiber that you eat. It has been found through research that people that eat more fiber are less prone to forming a Hiatus Hernia. When you have Hiatus Hernia, you do not want to struggle with constipation.

   You need to avoid any type of straining, whether it's to push out stubborn stools or lift heavy items. These pressures show up quickly in your stomach and LES area making it more difficult to recover from Hiatus Hernia.

6. What you drink and the way you drink it is important. In the food section area, you will find a list of fruits to drink and eat. It is through juices that you will get faster relief from Hiatus Hernia since juice nutrients are absorbed faster into your blood.

7. Use the natural remedies listed in the chapter on natural remedies. These remedies, when used consistently over time, start regenerating and protecting your cells and tissues from continued degeneration.

8. Take the supplements listed. This helps you to give those nutrients to the weakened muscles in your LES. When you have a condition like a hiatus hernia, you need to increase your supplements and eat more fruits and vegetables. This will strengthen the muscles and tissues that are causing your hernia.

9. In all health programs, you need to do some exercises. If you want to live your life out like it should be then

you need to exercise. Exercising does not need to be complicated. See the suggested exercises or do your own. You need good circulation throughout your body and strong abdominal muscle to stop Hiatus Hernia from growing.

10. When you head to bed, you should use two pillows to elevate your head as you sleep. Or, you can elevate your bed at the headboard by six to eight inches, by putting wooden blocks on the legs. Do this only when you are also fighting acid reflux.

11. If you are overweight, you will be prone to hiatus hernia and acid reflux. Using the dietary recommendations in this book will help you lose some weight.

12. Take your time to eat. Chew your food well. Eat small meals. When you eat a large amount of food, it will stay in your esophagus and stomach longer and stretch it. Don't overwork your esophagus and stomach by eating more than you should.

Practices to Avoid

Skip large meals and eat four small meals a day so that you don't over stress your stomach. You need to limit the work your stomach does, while you get rid of your Hiatus Hernia. When you have gotten relief from your hernia, you can eat three meals a day, using the new diet you have developed from this book.

After you eat, wait about two to three hours before you lie down or do any exertions.

Avoid eating spicy foods and if you take digestive enzymes use only those that do not have hydrochloric acid, HCl. If you have any inflammation or broken tissue in the esophagus, this food and HCl will aggravate these areas.

Don't eat fatty or fried foods, since they delay digestion and keep your food in the stomach longer.

Other things to avoid are coffee, black tea, alcohol, colas, sugary drinks, milk, junk food and smoking.

Make sure you are not eating food that you are allergic to. If you do, this will prolong your healing process.

If you have constipation, all the recommendation in this e-book will help you eliminate Hiatus Hernia and constipation.

Follow many of these recommendations and you will see not only a cure for Hiatus Hernia but a big improvement in your health. It will be worth it since you will learn some of the secrets of how to gain and maintain excellent health that you can use the rest of your life.

6: How to Test for an Acid Body

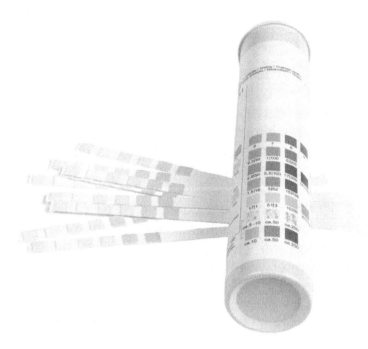

Saliva Test

If you want to get rid of hiatus hernia or acid reflux, you need to move your body to a more alkaline condition. You might think that you don't have an acid body, but if you are struggling with acid reflux or hiatus hernia, you definitely do.

Here is a simple test you can perform on your saliva that will give you an idea of where you stand with your body pH level. Your saliva contains mineral salts that keep it alkaline at 7.4. If your body is deficient in alkaline food or minerals, it will take these minerals from your saliva causing it to become more acidic.

If your saliva is below normal, you can influence your saliva's pH to read higher, by eating more acid binding (acid binding food will be explained in the next chapter) food and to supplement with potassium, magnesium, and calcium.

Keep in mind there are some inaccuracies with this test method since your body fluids are always in transition. This test simply gives you an idea of what your saliva pH is at that moment. Use this information for your own education. Then as you begin to change your eating habits and lifestyle, you can retest to see if there is a difference.

Many doctors deny the accuracy or use of this saliva test and say it is of no value. Some doctors say that many natural remedies are of no value unless approved by the FDA. Frankly, they prefer you to pay them a visit so that they can put you under their care, but, in an article written by Dr. Steven Zodkoy, A Free and Simple Test for pH, a Potential Health Tester, he promotes the use of this saliva pH test.

By testing your pH regularly, you can decide the validity of using pH litmus paper to determine the level of your health. As you make changes, you can test your saliva to see if the pH litmus color changes.

You need to take this test for 3 days and at least 3 times a day and get an average value so that you can establish a baseline or a starting point for yourself.

Purchase some pH litmus paper at a drug store, laboratory outlet or order it through the Internet. The better pH paper you can buy it on Amazon, with a .25 increment in pH change. Buy the litmus paper that is strips rather than rolls.

Starting Your Saliva Testing

Gather saliva in your mouth then swallow. Do this three times.

Place the pH paper under your tongue. Let it sit there for 5 seconds to wet it and then remove it. Let it sit for 10 seconds, compare the color of your pH paper to the color chart on the bottle, and record the pH.

Do this test around one hour before eating or around two hours after eating. This reading gives you an idea about the state of your saliva. Your first test should be done first thing in the morning before you rinse out your mouth or drink anything.

Saliva and Lemon Test

Now, do this test immediately after you do your saliva test above.

- Squeeze the juice of half a lemon into one ounce of water
- Swish it around in your mouth for 5 seconds
- Spit it out, wait one minute
- Place litmus paper into your mouth and wet it.
- Measure your mouth's pH and record the value.

Now compare the color and pH value of this reading with your first pH saliva reading. This reading should have a higher alkaline reading than your first saliva reading.

Good Saliva Test

If this reading has a higher alkaline value, than your first saliva reading, it means you have good alkaline reserves. You have plenty of minerals to help you neutralize the acids in your body.

The higher the alkaline reading you have the stronger your alkaline reserves. A small alkaline upward change means you have alkaline reserves, but they are not as strong as they should be.

For example,

- Morning reading is 6.5 pH (the higher the better)
- After the lemon test reading 6.9 pH

These readings are good and indicate you have somebody mineral stores. But your Morning reading of 6.5 is a little low and should be closer to 7.0 for better health.

Weak Saliva Test

If your pH reading does not change from your first reading or actually goes down by becoming more acidic, then your alkaline reserves are weak, and you need to make some major changes in the way you eat. In this course, you will see what you will need to do to bring up your alkaline reserves so that you will not be susceptible to serious diseases.

Now, suppose your readings were,

- First reading 6.5
- Lemon test reading 6.2

There is a drop in your lemon pH, and this is not too good. This means that you don't have enough minerals in your body to neutralize the acid in your mouth. You will have to eat more acid binding food.

Saliva Test Summary

Again, if your lemon test readings have a higher pH reading than your first reading, it means you have alkaline reserves. The bigger the difference between your first test and second test, the stronger your alkaline reserves. A small alkaline upward change means you have alkaline reserves, but they are not as strong as they should be.

If your lemon pH reading does not change from your first reading or actually goes down by becoming more acidic, then your alkaline reserves are weak. Because of this, you need to make some major changes in the way you eat. This also means you have a highly acidic body that can create some serious illness, especially if your lemon test pH is down to 6.0 and below.

Compute the pH Average

After three or four days of saliva, you want to take the average of all readings. Here is how you can determine what your pH readings mean.

- pH level of 6.5 to 7.4 - You are at a healthy level. However, the higher number is better.
- pH level of 6.0 to 6.5 – You may not be feeling good and need to make some changes in your diet.

- pH level of 5.0 to 6.0 - You have major health problems.

- pH level of 4.5 – 5.0 – You have a terminal disease.

Strive For This pH

You are considered to have an alkaline body if your overall body pH liquids are 6.5 to 7.4. This is the pH level that you should strive for. Higher pH values of 7.5 to 8.5 and up are considered detrimental.

Children with an acid body will respond quickly to good changes in eating habits, whereas adults, depending on age, can see results in 5 weeks and up to a year.

pH and Oxygen

Another important issue related to pH is the oxygen level. Tissue and cells have more oxygen available to them when your body pH is 7.4 as compared to when it is 6.4.

It has been found that the average American's tissue pH is between 5.5 and 6.0. This indicates that they have a severe lack of oxygen in their cells and lymph liquid. Lack of oxygen in the body is known to create serious terminal diseases. It is oxygen that destroys all types of bacteria and pathogens that live inside your body and make you ill.

Those of you with acid bodies and that lack cell and lymph oxygen can correct your condition by learning what it takes to bring your body back to an alkaline level. This will give your body a chance to repair tissue and organs, provided, they have not been severely damaged.

5: Eliminate An Acid Body-Create An Alkaline Body

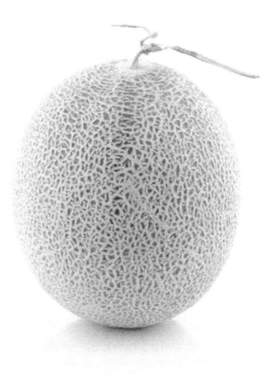

An Acid Body

Understanding acid and alkaline body condition is a critical concept to understand and use. It is this concept that turns any disease around.

An acid body is the worst condition you can have when you have hiatus hernia. An acid body is condition where body acids dominate and are slowly causing a deterioration of tissue, muscles, and organs. This deterioration gives rise to various body conditions that eventually lead to diseases that are hard to eliminate.

So your challenge, when you have an acid body is to change it to an alkaline body. Disease and pathogens do not like an alkaline body. Do you suffer from various pains in your body? If yes, then you have an acid body, and most people do.

If you have an acid body, it will take time to make your body alkaline. There are many things you need to do to create an alkaline body. Here is what you need to do,

- Eat more alkalizing food
- Eat less acid food
- Neutralize existing body acid and waste
- Neutralize daily acids that enter the body
- Neutralize acids produced by cell metabolism
- Neutralize acids created by body exercise
- Neutralize acids created by negative thinking
- Neutralize acids created by illness

Moving your body more toward alkalinity is what will help you with your hiatus hernia.

Mineral Food

The minerals you need to make your body alkaline are sodium, potassium, calcium, phosphorus, and magnesium. These minerals bind with acid so that they can be eliminated through your elimination channels. All of these minerals need to come from food and supplements. These minerals are called *acid binding minerals.*

Acid Binding

Acid-binding minerals are found in high quantities in fruits and vegetables. These minerals are sodium, potassium, calcium, magnesium, and phosphorus. What acid binding means is when you eat fruits with these minerals, they will combine with acids in your body and neutralize them. These neutralized acids will be then be eliminated from your body, in your urine and feces.

So you can see the importance of getting a lot of acid-binding minerals into your body. Without them, acids would not get eliminated, from your body. They would remain in your body tissues and continue their bodily damage.

Alkaline Binding

Now, there is another side to this story. You have acid binding, and you have alkaline binding. There are minerals that become alkaline binding. These minerals are sulfur, iodine, phosphorus, bromine, fluorine, copper, and silicon. These minerals when digested by a cell will produce a salt that will bind with acid binding minerals (the alkalizing minerals) and eliminate them from your body.

When alkaline minerals are trapped by an acid salt, the alkaline mineral is removed from your body, and your body becomes more acidic. This is the condition you are trying to avoid.

The Foods that are alkaline binding and remove the minerals that you need to make your body alkaline are meat, carbohydrates, junk food, all food in packages and cans and some vegetables and some fruits.

Acid Thoughts

Now, we have talked about acid toxins in your body that are brought in through food and the environment. But, there are other factors that create acid in your body, and these are emotions that are activated through life stresses, work pressures, divorce, friendship problems, marital issues, and other similar situations.

These emotional problems create acidic molecules that embed themselves into your tissues just like food acids. These acid molecules can be neutralized with minerals.

Acid Binding Foods

Here is a list of the fruits that have the highest acid binding minerals and the ones that you should be eating to eliminate your body's acids.

The percentage assigned to these fruits is based on fresh fruits that are organic, and that they are not cooked, canned or mixed with sugar.

Fruits above 50% in value are more acid binding, which means they will trap acid wastes better. You will want to eat and drink more of those fruits that are above 51%.

The fruits that are at 50% at are neutral. They are not acid binding nor alkaline binding.

Here is the list of fruits and vegetables to eat and drink in the order of priority.

Fruits that Bind Acid

1. **Fruits at 100% Acid Binding** – Best fruits To Eat
   Lemons, melons – any type, watermelon

2. **Fruits at 93% Acid Binding** – great fruits To Eat
   Cantaloupes, dried dates, dried figs, limes, mango, papaya

3. **Fruits at 87% Acid Binding** – still Great Fruits To Eat.
   Kiwis, passion fruit, pineapples, raisins, umeboshi plums

4. **Fruits at 80% Acid Binding** – eat These Fruits
   Apricots, avocados, bananas, fresh dates, fresh figs, currants, gooseberries, grapes, grapefruits, guavas, kumquats, nectarines, pears, persimmons, quince, berries, cactus

5. **Fruits at 73% Acid Binding** – still Fruits To Eat
   Apples, oranges, peaches, pomegranate, raspberries, sour grapes, strawberries, carob

6. **Fruits at 67% Acid Binding** – still Neutralizes Acids
   Cherries, fresh coconut

Other Foods that are Acid Binding

7. **Herbal Teas From Leaves at 73% to 86% acid binding**

Alfalfa, mint, sage, spearmint, raspberry strawberry comfrey

8. All Herbs and Spices at 67% to 73% Acid Binding

Fruits At 40% to 47% Alkaline Binding - eat less of these fruits

Blueberries, cranberries, plums, prunes

Vegetables that Bind Acids

Here is the list of vegetables to eat in order of priority. All of these vegetables will neutralize acid, since they contain minerals that are acid binding.

9. Vegetables at 93% Acid Binding – best vegetables to eat

Kelp, Seaweed, Watercress, Asparagus

10. Vegetables at 80% Acid Binding – still the best to eat

Lettuce Leaf, Oyster plant, Pumpkin, Spinach, Squash, Peas, Carrots, Celery, Chard, Swiss, Dandelion greens

11. Vegetables at 73% Acid Binding – great vegetables to eat

Bamboo shoots, Beets, Broccoli, Cabbage, Cauliflower, Collards, Corn, sweet, Ginger (fresh), Mushrooms,

Mustard greens, Onions, Pepper, Potatoes, Green, Lima, String, Potatoes

12. **Vegetables at 67% Acid Binding** – eat plenty of these Brussel sprouts, Cucumbers, Eggplants, Okra, Onions, Radishes, Tomatoes

13. **Vegetable juices at 80% to 93% Acid Binding** - Parsley, wheatgrass, carrot, celery, etc.

14. **Soy Bean Products at 60% Acid Binding** – limit your use of tofu since it is a genetically modified organism, GMO Dried beans, Soy cheese, Soy milk, Tempeh, Tofu

Misc. Acid Binding Food

1. Starches at 80% Acid Binding

Arrowroot flour

Sugar   at   73%   acid   Binding

Honey

2. Nuts and Seeds at 60 % to 67% Acid Binding

Almonds, sesame seeds, Granola, Essene Bread, Chestnuts

3. Misc.   foods   at   60%   Acid   Binding

Horseradish, Amaranth, Millet, Quinoa, Dried beans, Soy cheese, Soy milk,

NOTE: The lower the alkaline binding percentage, the more the food produces acid in your body.

4. All oils are basically at 50% and are considered neutral.

This includes almond, avocado, canola, coconut, corn castor, olive, soy, sunflower oil.

5. Beans, starches, and nuts and seeds are at 40% to   46%   Alkaline   Binding

Aduki, Black, Broadbean, Garbanzo, Mung, Pinto, Barley, Corn Meal, Lentils, Brans, Cashews, Coconut (dried), Pecans, Brans, Millet, Filberts, Walnuts, Pumpkin, Sunflower

6. Starches are at 26 to 33 % Alkaline Binding

Brown Rice, Buckwheat, Oats, Spelt, Wheat Whole, Peanuts, corn, rye

7. Rice   at   20%   Alkaline   Binding

White rice

8. Sugar   at   13%   Alkaline   Binding

White beet or cane sugar

Meat and Fish that Are Alkaline binding

9. Meat   at   26%   alkaline   binding

Fish With fins and scales, Shellfish - shrimp, scallops, crab lobster, oyster

10. Meat   at   20%   Alkaline   Binding

Chicken, turkey, rabbit

11. Meat   at   13%   Alkaline   Binding

Beef, goat, pork, lamb

12. All oils are basically at 50% and are considered neutral.

This includes almond, avocado, canola, coconut, corn castor, olive, soy, sunflower oil.

13. Misc. Products at 13% to 26% Alkaline Binding

Liquor, wine, beer, coffee, black tea, caffeine drinks

You should be eating 80% acid binding foods and 20% alkaline binding foods. When you eat with this 80/20 formula, you will have an alkaline body, over a period of time. Just gradually work toward this formula.

These are the basic eating principle you should use to achieve ultimate health.

7: Body Cycle That Can Fix Hiatus Hernia

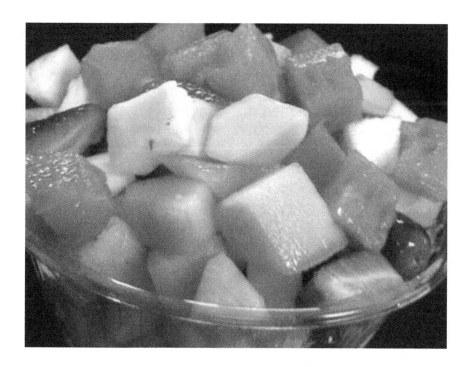

Natural Body Cycles

Most people don't know about body cycles. The body has various cycles where it does certain body processes and it does these processes every day. Here is the basis of how you can assist your body cycles to strengthen your whole body and to set the stage for eliminating your Hiatus Hernia.

If you are overweight, following the body cycle will help you lose some pounds. If you have constipation or flatulence, the body cycle, when allowed to work, will reduce this issue for you. Here is what you need to do to help your body perform their body cycles. What this requires is a new way of what you eat and when you do it. Following these techniques will surely improve your overall health.

Since all of us are addicted to the way we eat, it is, sometimes, difficult to change these habits. But if you are serious about what you want, this is the best information that will give you good health.

By using this method to gain better health, you will experience side effects because you will be eliminating more body toxins and body wastes. The side effects may be headaches, stomach upsets, body pain, or similar types of symptoms. These conditions will not last and will disappear as you get rid of more toxins.

Here are the 3 natural body cycles:

Cycle 1 time period: 4 a.m. to 12 noon

This cycle is the time where your body is eliminating toxins, acids, wastes, and derby by urine, bowel movements, and other secretions.

During the elimination cycle, 4 a.m. to 12 noon, eat and drink only fruits and their juices or drink vegetable juices. For breakfast eat a bowl of fruit or have a fruit smoothie made with apple juice and fruits in season. Before noontime, you should eat fruit as a snack. Forty-five minutes before noon, eat your last fruit. You can eat and drink all the fruits and juices you want up to noontime.

By eating in this way you are assisting your body's elimination cycle. This helps your body to eliminate toxins and acids from your body and blood. It is these toxins and acids that make you sick and overweight and weaken your LES. Acids are the main cause of most illnesses, and so you want to have an alkaline body. Fruits and vegetables give you an alkaline body.

It takes one hour or so to digest fruit and fruit juices. Because of this, they help to cleanse your body of waste. Fruits are 70% water just like your body, and this gives them the cleansing action they have and that your body needs.

Cycle 2 time period: 12 noon to 8 p.m.

This is the time when your body should be taking in food and digesting. During this period is time to eat solid food. What you eat has to be in alignment with what your stomach can do. Your stomach can only work on one solid food at a time, so your lunch and dinner should only have one solid food. A lunch can consist of chicken and a green salad, fish and a green salad, tuna and a green salad, shrimp and a green salad, beef and a green salad.

Any eating habit that disrupts cycle 2, the eating and digestion cycle, affects the other cycles. Here's how you can help your body's cycle 2 to be more effective.

1. Eat only one solid food with vegetables during lunch or dinner. Lunch can be one meat or seafood with a fresh vegetable salad.

2. Limit the amount of water you drink during your eating. Excess water will dilute your digestive acids and slow down digestion of your food. It may even cause you to have an incomplete digestion of protein.

3. Eliminate drinking any sodas, coffee, tea or other drinks during your meals. If you need to clear your dry throat use a little water, which is a room temperature. Cold liquids will slow down your digestive processes. This will take a little bit of persistent to learn this habit, but it will pay off for you in the long run.

4. Eating meals with more than one solid food such as meat and potatoes, chicken and rice, fish and rice, chicken and noodles, eggs and toast, cheese and bread will diminish the energy you need during the elimination cycle 1.

5. It is permissible to eat beef and chicken at the same time but not chicken and eggs or beef and nut or chicken and beans. Eat the same type of protein at the same time but do not mix different proteins.

6. Its ok to eat different types of carbohydrates at the same time, with a salad, but not with protein, since carbohydrates digest easier than protein.

Eating the right combinations of foods at mealtime helps to preserve your energy for the elimination cycle and prevents you from creating spoiled food in your stomach that is converted to acid waste. It is this acid waste that results in illness and fat. This is the reason most people as they age come down with various illnesses that terminate their lives early.

Cycle 3 time period: 8 p.m. to 4 a.m.

This is the time your body is absorbing and using the food you have eaten during the noon to 8 p.m. period. This is the time the food you have eaten during the day is assimilated, absorbed and distributed throughout your body through your blood. Food that was eaten during body cycle II, and that was combined and eaten properly will digest within three hours. A meal consisting of protein and carbohydrates will take up to eight hours to pass through the stomach. During this time, your food will putrefy and ferment and become acidic with an increase stomach pressure. Under these conditions, you will not get the most nutrients from that meal.

Eat your last meal by 6-7pm so that your food digests in your stomach by the time you go to bed. Three hours later, your food will have moved into your small intestine where it is ready for assimilation. When you go to bed three hours after your last meal, the next six hours, until 4 am, your body will be absorbing the food you have eaten the previous day and removing waste and placing them in the urine and feces.

Remember, anything you do differently than what these cycles call for will disrupt them and cause them to become extended. When this happens, your food turns into acid, you don't absorb the value of your food, you lose energy and become tired, and over time, you gain weight and create serious illnesses.

8: Food You Should Eat To Fix Hiatus Hernia

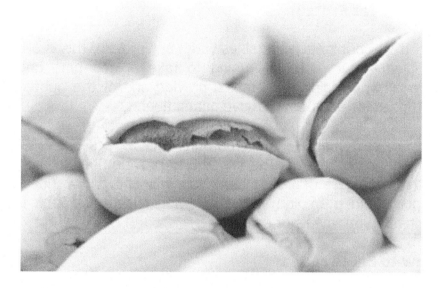

It is best to eat smaller meals when you eat. You may want to eat four meals per day. The smaller meals allow your stomach to process this food easier, giving your stomach less stress. Your stomach will have a chance to digest your food better and create more nutrients for your cells and tissues.

There are certain foods that are more detrimental to your health than others. For this reason, you should minimize eating these foods. Here are some eating guidelines to use.

Eat less protein and bread

Protein stays in your stomach for up to four hours, since it takes a long time to digest. If you don't have enough stomach acid, some of the protein you eat will not get digested. So having good stomach acid, less than 2.5 will give good protein digestion. When you don't digest protein like you should, bad bacteria will thrive in your colon. Bad bacteria live on undigested protein.

How to Eat Protein

If you don't eat vegetables with your protein, this is a big problem. Your protein is going to take a long time going through your colon. Vegetables provide one of the nutrients you need for good bowel movements, fiber.

So, eat smaller protein portions and always eat it with some raw vegetables. The vegetables provide fiber to mix in with the digested protein and you will know why fiber is important in the colon in the following chapters. Don't eat fruit with your meals or as dessert.

How to Eat Bread

Now, the same is true about bread or other white flour products. They digest quicker than protein in the stomach, but in the colon, they move very slowly. Again, eat them with vegetables unless you want to have or keep your constipation.

When's the Best Time to Eat Protein and Carbohydrates?

Now, here is the best way to eat protein and carbohydrates. At lunch or dinner only eat one or the other with raw vegetables. Cooked vegetables can be ok if you only cook them for a few minutes and with a little water. If you can do it, eat protein and vegetables and no carbohydrates. Or, eat carbohydrates and vegetables and no protein. And, again eat fruits and their juices only in the morning. But you can eat them as afternoon snacks or about 1 1/2 hour after meals.

Dairy products are associated with constipation. This includes milk, cream soups, cheese, yogurt, and some desserts and baked goods.

The best dairy product to eat is cottage cheese. It is the least harmful to the body of all dairy products.

Food Not To Eat

Your colon is designed to move undigested matter and various bodily wastes through its tract and out your rectum. It does this naturally only when this matter and waste have bulk or fiber and water. It is this bulk or fiber that pushes against your colon walls and triggers peristaltic action. You can only get this bulk to the right consistency when you eat plenty of fruits, vegetables, and grains that have a combination of soluble and non-soluble fiber.

Processed food, meat, fish, and dairy products have little or no fiber. In your colon, these foods do not move easily and remain too long in your colon.

Processed foods are stripped of fiber and a lot of their nutrients. They get into your bloodstream quickly and flood your blood with excess sugar. These foods contain various un-natural chemicals that your liver sees as toxic and tries to store them somewhere in your body so that they don't harm you.

Vitamin Enhanced Food

It doesn't matter if the manufacturer put back some vitamins into their processed food. This food is still not healthy and is an unbalanced food. Only natural foods are balanced and do no harm.

Processed foods are those foods that come in a package such as a bag, box, a can, or plastic bottle. Any of these foods are unhealthy if eaten long term.   When sick it is best to avoid these foods, since they require your vitamins, minerals, and enzymes to fully digest and absorb them.

All bottle juices or canned fruits and vegetables have had their digestive enzymes destroyed by heat and pressure. When you eat these foods, you have to provide the enzymes to digest them. When you have to provide digestive enzymes for processed foods, you decrease your lifespan, and you alter the good health that you can have.

Foods Not to Eat

You need to stay away from foods that aggravate your acid reflux or hiatus hernia. These foods vary from person to person, but here is a list that is known to cause stomach problems:

- Tomato based foods
- Onions
- Garlic
- Fried foods, fatty meats,
- Citrus fruits, grapefruit, lemon, cranberry juices
- Chocolate or cocoa
- Caffeine
- Alcohol, wine, beer
- Caffeine
- Artificial sweeteners

- Canola oil
- Excess salt
- Processed foods, foods in packages or cans
- Whole milk
- Peppermint
- Cottage cheese
- Ice cream
- Spicy foods, but test cayenne pepper to see if it help you

You may have a longer or shorter list. Once you have improved or eliminated your hiatus condition, you can again eat some of these foods. But you have to test to see which ones still give you problems.

Foods to Eat

- leafy greens lettuces
- carrots and broccoli
- Green beans
- Apples and bananas
- species, ginger, cinnamon, coriander, cardamom
- whole nuts and seeds
- green tea non-caffeinated
- lean protein, skinless chicken, turkey, fish, lean beef, or pork
- whole grains

- non-citrus fruits or juices, if not tolerated
- Fermented foods such as:
- pickles, kefir, cheese, kimchi sauerkraut, kombucha
- unsweetened yogurt, buttermilk, skim milk
- fat-free cheese
- bake or broil food
- skim off fat from cooking meat
- use seasoning in moderation
- steam vegetables
- limit butter, cream sauces, oils and cooking sprays

Anti-oxidants

All vegetables and fruits contain hundreds of chemicals called anti-oxidants. It is these chemicals that tie up and eliminate free radicals. You need to consume as many of these anti-oxidants as possible. These chemicals reduce the inflammation that occurs when you have hiatal hernia. By reducing inflammation, you enhance your immune system and give it more power to fix your hernia.

Vegetables To Eat

One of the ways to maintain better health is to eat more fruits and vegetables. There is just no way around this. The purpose of eating more produce is to detoxify and maintain your body in an alkaline condition and to provide the nutrients needed throughout your body to keep you in good health.

What vegetables and fruits do is bring more oxygen into your body and all organs. It makes your body alkaline. It is well known now that when your body fluids are acidic, you will be prone to more illness and disease. First of all, acid in your body creates inflammation. Low-grade inflammation, that you don't feel slowly leads to the deterioration of organs and tissue.

That is why as your year's pass, you can start to see the appearance of various diseases in your body. Second various pathogens like an acid environment and set up household in your body. As these pathogens, bacteria, viruses, and parasite multiple, they make your body more acidic because of their excretions.

Pathogens don't like an alkaline environment. Here is how you can start to make your body more alkaline. First, you need to get in tune with your body cycles, and then you need to eat more fruits and vegetables. This will be a start. There are many more natural things to do, but making these changes is a great start in changing the way you feel and reducing the illnesses you would create.

Citrus fruits may cause some you some problems. But if they don't, then you can include them in your diet.

Citrus Fruits

Most people see citrus fruits - grapefruits, oranges, lemons, and limes – as acid food. The secret of citrus is that even though they enter your mouth as an acid food they work in your body as an alkaline residue. This residue works to eliminate acid, which makes you less susceptible to disease.

Grapefruit

Nutritionally, grapefruit is high in vitamin C and contains flavonoids different from the other citrus fruits. On its skin, the grapefruit has a phytochemical called monoterpenes, which has been found to protect against cancer. Very few people eat the skin since it is quite bitter. However, these skin phytochemicals lower blood cholesterol and clean out arterial plaque.

This could be a natural remedy to reverse atherosclerosis. Most people just eat the meat of the grapefruit, but the rind has been found, in Japan, to be high in vitamins and in nutrients that fight cancer.

The rind is also bitter, but you always get a little when you peel the grapefruit. The skin of the grapefruit can be cut into bite-size pieces and dried on your counter. After a week or two, you can store them in a glass jar and chew on them when you have an upset stomach.

Lemons and Antioxidants

Lemons go way back to 800 B.C. Now, lemons have monoterpenes like grapefruit. These monoterpenes are powerful antioxidants, and in combination with vitamin C have cancer prevention and fighting abilities.

Lemons are considered acidic but when their nutrients enter the body and are used up, the residue becomes alkaline. This residue becomes available to neutralize body acids. Most people have acid bodies and lack minerals to adjust their bodies back to normal or alkaline.

So, lemons and other citric fruits should be eaten daily, even if you have arthritis.

Limes and Monoterpenes

Limes have similar properties as lemons since they too contain monoterpenes. You can eat the outer skin to get the most health benefit from limes. Throw them in a blender with other juices to get a strong citrus drink.

Oranges and D-limonene

Oranges existed in China in 2400 B.C. Through trading, oranges were spread throughout Europe and the rest of the world. Oranges are high in vitamin C, and their skin contains a good amount of monoterpenes and oil called d-limonene. Use citrus fruits daily for their vitamin C, phytonutrients, and antioxidants that protect you from cancer and other diseases. Use them for arthritis to neutralize and remove acids that surround joints and cause inflammation.

9: Fiber For Your Hiatus Hernia Recovery

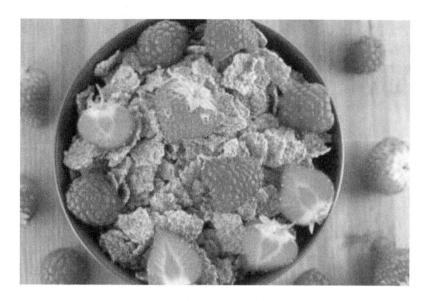

What is Fiber?

One of the main reasons you might have hiatus hernia is that you don't have enough fiber in your diet. Fiber is a necessary substance that prevents you from having constipation. When you have frequent constipation and you strain to have a bowel movement, you put pressure on the top of your stomach, which can force it into your upper diaphragm. The result is hiatus hernia.

Fiber is a carbohydrate that comes from the cell's walls and structure of plants, grains, legumes, fruits, and vegetables. Most processed or junk food has little or no fiber, which was removed during processing.

Most people eat around 7-12 grams of fiber each day. You should be eating from 25 – 40 grams each day to prevent serious illnesses in your body.

A diet with 40 grams of fiber provides protection and prevention against diseases such as kidney stones, varicose veins, obesity, heart disease, appendicitis, colon disease, diabetes, appendicitis, diverticulosis, and conditions such as Hiatus Hernia.

It will be difficult for you to reach 40 grams of fiber a day if you are not eating very man fruits and vegetables. So you have to start adding produce to your diet slowly so your body does not give you side effects.

When you eat fiber, it passes into your colon without getting digested in the small intestine. The good bacteria will use some of it as food, which makes them stronger and able to multiply.

Eating fiber reduces your fecal matter transit time from three days to 1 1/ 2 - 2days.

All processed foods, such as white flour products, have little or no fiber. Fiber is removed when various natural flours or grains are processed to make junk food. During this processing, nutrients, vitamins, and minerals are also removed. Only plant foods and lightly processed grains have fiber of varying amounts.

Soluble Fiber

Soluble Fiber becomes gummy and viscous, after it dissolves in water.

Soluble fiber can slow down digestion in the small intestine and prevent simple sugars from entering the bloodstream right away.

Because it absorbs water, soluble fiber softens and gives weight to fecal matter, and this makes fecal matter easier to pass through your colon.

Soluble fiber consists of pectin, gum, and mucilage. Pectin is found in carrots, apples, beets, cabbage, citrus fruits, and bananas. Gums and mucilage are found in oat bran, sesame seeds, oats, oatmeal, legumes, guar gum, and gum Arabic

Insoluble Fiber

Insoluble fiber does not dissolve in water and consists of cellulose, hemicellulose, and lignin. This type of fiber is extremely beneficial to your health. Because your body's enzymes cannot break down this fiber, like it does food, it remains in tack as it travels through your intestines and colon.

Insoluble fiber helps fecal matter travel faster through the small intestine and your colon. It provides bulk to your fecal matter. It makes your stools larger, softer, and stimulates peristaltic movement as it touches your colon walls.

Insoluble fibers are found in vegetables, wheat, and wheat bran. This type of fiber is considered an anti-carcinogen and a digestive aid. It is credited with preventing colon cancer and many other colon diseases.

Eating Fiber

As you can see, fiber is a critical nutrient for your colon

and overall health. You need to eat equal amounts of insoluble and soluble fiber. Most people only eat around 10 grams or less of fiber each day. The amount you need to eat is around 25 – 40 grams. This is a lot of fiber, and you will need to introduce it slowly into your diet. You may experience gas when you eat more fiber than you normally do.

Health Alert: If you have any serious gastrointestinal illnesses, check with your doctor before adding more fiber to your diet.

If you have not been eating a lot of fiber in the form of vegetable, fruits, and grains, you need to add these foods to your eating habits little by little so your body gets used to more fiber.

Health Tip: Provide yourself with natural forms of fiber, such as vegetables, fruits, and legumes. Stay away from the supplemental forms of fiber such as, powders or pills that may help in relieving constipation but do little to provide you with other nutrients those natural forms of fiber provide.

Eating Bran

Eating bran is one of the quickest and best ways to increase your fiber. It will increase the weight and size of your stools more than the fiber contained in fruits or vegetables. Bran is the outer husk of the grain – wheat, corn, rice, and oat – which is indigestible.

Use one or two heaping tablespoons of bran in your morning cereal, in your baking, and in your smoothies.

Health Alert: When using bran, make sure you drink plenty of water during the day to keep your stools soft.

There are four basic bran products – wheat, corn, oat, and rice. They all provide a solid source of fiber in varying amounts. Make sure the bran you use is 100% unprocessed bran. Here are the two recommended bran products.

Oat Bran

Oat bran has both soluble and insoluble fiber, which make it better to use than wheat bran. However, it does have less insoluble fiber than wheat and rice bran. It can be found with relatively little processing, which helps to maintain its high quality of protein, carbohydrates, and vitamins.

Rice Bran

For preventing constipation, rice bran is better than wheat bran. Do not take your calcium supplement with bran cereals, since fiber can interfere with calcium absorption.

Do not use cereal with bran in it. This bran has been processed and loses some of its fiber content. Use the bran sold as coarse granules. Add it to your morning cereals, smoothies, shakes, cottage cheese, yogurt, or other dishes.

Sources of Insoluble Fiber

- Bananas
- Broccoli
- Brown rice
- Brussels sprouts
- Cauliflower
- Cabbage

- Corn
- Lentils
- Potatoes
- Spinach wheat germ
- Whole wheat bread
- Whole wheat crackers

Sources of Soluble Fiber

Oranges, grapefruit, nectarines, peaches, tangerines, apples, berries, apricots, bananas, figs, prunes

Zucchini, turnips, okra, cabbage, peas, sweet potatoes

Carrots, celery, broccoli, cauliflower, corn, eggplant, okra, Zucchini, greens

Barley, chickpeas, split peas, pinto beans, kidney beans, navy beans, potatoes

10: What To Drink To Stop Hiatus Hernia

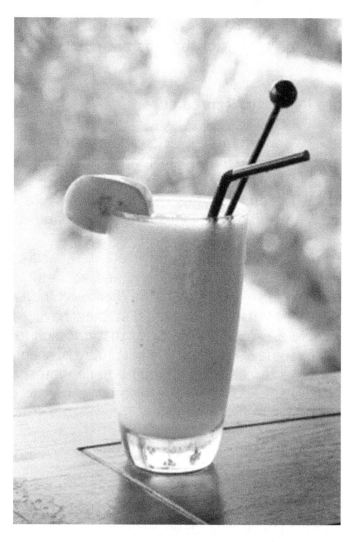

Here are some of the best fruits juices that you need to drink for Hiatus Hernia. If you can, use organic fruits and make your own fresh juices. If it is not possible, then buy only fruit juices in bottle containers.

Use them between meals, before a meal, in some cases, or just before bedtime. You can also drink the juices that are listed in the previous lessons that are not listed here. The important thing is you can target certain juices for a specific illness, or use them as a general body tonic. Use a variety of juices to get the benefit of the different nutrients that these fruit juices have.

Juices are Powerful Remedies

Juices are powerful remedies and sources of quick health. They are concentrated in their nutrients and are quickly, within minutes, absorbed into your blood, since they require little or no digestion. For this reason, you can use them to rebuild, cleanse, and detoxify your body quickly and easily.

Juices can help you prevent, retard, or cure illness. However, they must be used properly and at the right times. In some cases, use of juices as a therapy can have side effects, but when used in moderation they have little side effects. There are certain fruit juices that are high in natural sugars, so if you have diabetes it is best to avoid them. If you have a sensitive throat or a respiratory issue, you should not use citrus juices. And, there are also some people that are allergic to specific fruits.

Diseases and Juices

All diseases respond to the use of specific fruit juices because they correct and rebalance the heat or cold in the body. They remove and neutralize toxins. So, use them when you have a fever or when you have a cold.

At times, juices can pull out too many toxins from your body, if you are too toxic causing you to feel sick and uneasy.

Some people get an upset stomach if they drink juices as the first thing in the morning. I suspect that this happens because juices are detoxifying the stomach and gastrointestinal tract. Juice Side effects can range from headaches to rashes or pain. Side effects will subside as you drink the juices and continue to detoxify your body.

Fresh juices are easy to create with a juicer and give you the pleasure of knowing you are giving your body the nutrients it needs.

Always drink fresh juice when possible. One glass of juice can count as more than one serving of fruit. Bottled juice no longer has the pH that fresh juice has and loses a slight amount of its pH value. However, when certain juices are not available fresh, it is always best to use bottled or packaged juice to preserve your health. Avoid buying juices in cans, aluminum containers, and plastic bottles. These juices have been highly processed and tend to have reduced nutritional value.

Start Drinking Juices

Papayas

Papaya juice is a highly curative fruit, and its juice gives a powerful punch for health. It keeps arteries soft and flexible, preventing the deposition of cholesterol. Its digestive enzyme, pepsin, destroys the outer layer of germs, including the TB bacteria. It reduces the risk of high blood pressure, heart attacks, and improves the circulation of blood, improves liver function, restores peristaltic intestinal action, and improves vision. It is good for the aged, since it will improve their digestion allowing more nutrients to get into their body. It is a powerful meat digestive enzyme.

Mango Juice

Mango is another health winner. Its juice helps to build muscles and to strengthen tissues that are needed when you have Hiatus Hernia. It is an excellent heart and brain tonic. It is useful in constipation, digestive issues, reducing phlegm and acidity. It can expel worms, acts as an aphrodisiac, and blood rejuvenator and purifier.

Mango juice will improve vitality; It helps you gain weight and tones your nervous system. Using mango juice and milk will increase your red blood cell count. It will improve appetite, reduce constipation, and reduce insomnia when taken before bed time.

Here's how to use mango juice:

Mix one part milk with two parts mango juice or puree and four parts water.

Using mango juice in this fashion strengthens your immune system so it can fight off various conditions that can compromise your health. In addition, this mixture will help protect you from sun-stroke, nausea, and vomiting.

Apples

Because apples have a high mineral content, they are especially good for your skin, hair, and fingernails. Apples that are good for juices are Granny Smith, Braeburn, Egremont Russet, and Discovery. Gala apples are also good for juicing and eating. If they are firm and crisp, they provide good juice. When buying apple juice, buy juice that is cloudy and not clear. The cloudy juice has more fiber and nutrients and contains a good amount of the fiber pectin.

Apple juice serves as a good base when mixed with other juices and especially with vegetables. This will be covered in another lesson. Most of the vitamin A lies in the skin of the apple, so it is best to juice apples without peeling.

This is one of the fruits that can be used in many ways, and you still get it nutritional value. You can eat it raw, cooked, baked, juiced, jammed, or pickled.

Grape Juice

I usually add grape juice to other juices like apple to give it a different flavor. When juicing apples, juice a few handfuls of grape juice and mix them together. Grapes have a high content of natural sugar and can give you a quick energy lift. They contain a high level of minerals and have B vitamins. Many times I will drink this juice from bottles since it has a short season and in a bottle, you can drink it any time. Use the darker grape drinks, because of their high anti-oxidant nutrients

Grapes help to regulate and increase your metabolism. A low metabolism will cause you to gain weight, and a high metabolism will help you burn food quicker. Because of its mineral content, it helps to build your blood and to stimulate your liver to increase its cleansing abilities. The color of fruit juices often tells you what part of the body it is good for. Red grape juice helps build your blood.

Cherries

Fresh cherry juice is a powerful body alkalizer and reduces the acidity in your blood and tissues. It is an excellent remedy to reduce and eliminate gout pain and to make your body alkaline. Gout is an excess of acid in the joints and tissue. It is also good for prostate conditions. Drinking this juice between meals will help activate peristaltic bowel action, which can help to keep you regular.

Melons, Cantaloupes

All of the melons create super juices filled the best nutrient your body can use. They are at the top of the list for making your body more alkaline. They are good for your skin and provide your nerves nutrients. Melons have a cooling effect on the body and improve your digestion.

Watermelon

Watermelon juice can be obtained by simply eating raw watermelon since it is 98% distilled water. Its use helps cleanse the kidney and bladder since it is a diuretic – removes excess fluids from the body. You can chew down the seeds as you eat watermelon to get the extra zinc and vitamin E.

Watermelon juice tones your body prevents heat stroke, normalizes high blood pressure, and strengthens your heart and brain. It helps to cure jaundice and spleen enlargement. It improves digestion, cures chronic headaches, controls nausea and vomiting, calms the nerves, and is a mild laxative. This is one of the juices that will help you with Hiatus Hernia.

Eat watermelon in the morning to get its juice, which will help you remove nightly accumulated toxins through your urine. This will you restore kidney function.

Guava

Guava is hard to juice, but it can be bought as a juice. Guava is an excellent body cleanser. It helps to remove intestinal worms, eliminate constipation, improve digestion, and has aphrodisiac value. It strengthens the heart, improves blood circulation and is antiseptic.

You can buy guava juice, and in a blender mix it with pineapple juice and then add some fresh guava fruit to produce a highly effective body cleanser.

Pineapple Juice

Pineapple juice is another excellent juice to use frequently. Its high potassium, which helps to strengthen the muscles associated with the LES valve and helps to keep your nerve transmission active. Its health value comes from the enzyme bromelain that it contains. Bromelain helps keep body fluids balance and neutral; It moves an acid body to neutral and an alkaline one to neutral. It stimulates the pancreas to release its hormones. And, it has been found useful for coughs and sore throats. For some people, pineapple juice affects the throat making it feel scratchy.

When making pineapple juice do not juice the center core since it contains harmful chemicals. You can drink pineapple juice just before a meal as an appetizer. It helps to rejuvenate and cleanse your body. It also acts as a laxative so it helps to reduce constipation.

Try not to use pineapple juice on an empty stomach, since it could be harmful and can give you an upset stomach, because of the enzyme bromelain. You can drink it 10 – 15 minutes after a meal or when eating other fruits it is compatible with. It is a juice and fruit to be avoided by

pregnant women or women trying to get pregnant, since it contracts the uterus.

Pomegranate

Pomegranate juice controls bile and phlegm, increases hemoglobin and purifies blood, and improves appetite, and settles upset stomachs. It restores and sharpens memory, and is effective in urinary issues. It is helpful in many diseases since it neutralizes body acids. It will cure nosebleed by placing a couple drops in each nose. It is excellent for reducing fever. Drinking half a glass twice a day will help you reduce high blood pressure.

Vegetable Juices

Fresh vegetable juices have high nutritional, healing, and curing powers. Using vegetable juices as juice therapy has been used throughout the world for centuries, to help the body recover from nearly aliment. By separating the juice from its fiber, its minerals and nutrients are suspended in the distilled water of the juice. This allows for your body to digest and absorb vegetable juice within minutes as compared with hours when eating the entire vegetable.

Consider vegetable drinks as a meal. They should not be drunk with a meal or with any other food. You can add brewer's yeast, vitamin C powder, or acidophilus powder to them. You can take digestive enzymes with those juices that are not fresh and that come in a can, bottle, or are frozen.

Avoid those vegetable juices that are high in salt content. If you are drinking tomato juice, drink only that juice that is 100% tomato.

You can mix certain juices together to get a better taste. You can use the pulp from juicing vegetables to thicken soups or for a compost pile.

If you don't like to eat vegetables, or if you are sick and need to recover, then juicing is the ideal way to get nutrients into your body. Juicing vegetables is another way to get the benefits of vegetables without eating them. Juicing them does not get you the entire benefit of the whole vegetable.

Aloe Vera Juice

This juice is used for soothing the bowel area when it is irritated. If you have hemorrhoids, it can provide you some relief. Here's how to use it. There are some aloe vera juice drinks that you can buy at a health-food store. Try them out and see what your results are. If you have 98 to 99% aloe jell, mix 1-2 tablespoons with 7 up, some other carbonated drink or orange juice. Try different aloe portions until you find one that is palatable.

Aloe vera juice is also good if you have an ulcer or some internal lining scratch or tear. Aloe promotes the repair and regrowth of cells.
Go to a health-food store and buy some aloe vera juice. This juice is not 100% aloe. It has been diluted with juice.

Drink 1/4 to 1/2 a glass of Aloe Vera juice in the morning and evening.

Green Juices

Green drinks are a must. No matter what illness you have, you need to have a green drink. Even if don't have an illness, green drinks should be first on your list

A green drink can be used every day. Try to use a green drink at least twice a week. Using liquid chlorophyll is great, if you don't have a green drink. Squeeze the juice of one lemon into 1/2 oz. of chlorophyll then add 6 oz. of water. This can be drunk every-day first thing in the morning.

Blue-Green Manna is another powder you can use. It is high in chlorophyll and enzymes in the chlorophyll. This Manna is great for regulating the pancreas. You can check on the internet for capsules. You can add a couple of ounces of fresh pineapple, apple, and grape juice to make it more palatable. Adding a pinch of honey is another way to take a green drink.

Cabbage Juice

Cabbage juice is well known for curing duodenum ulcers and can even help esophageal ulcers, but it has a strong taste. Try combining it with carrot juice for a more palatable drink. It contains a substance called vitamin U, which is not really a vitamin.
It is vitamin U that gives cabbage juice its power to eliminate or cure stomach or duodenal ulcers. Heating cabbage or cabbage juice will destroy the vitamin U and its ability to relieve ulcers.

Drinking cabbage juice regularly can help you reduce nervousness, fear, depression, headaches, restlessness, and trembling, anxiety, and pessimistic views.

Drink 2 to 4 oz. of cabbage juice 4 to 5 times per day for up to 10 to 14 days.

Cabbage juice tends to create gas in the intestines. This is caused by the juice combining with putrefied matter and creating a gas. This is a natural process where this juice is performing a cleansing action in your body.

Carrot Juice

Carrot juice is the king of juices since it has so many health benefits and can be mixed with other juices to make them more palatable. It rejuvenates the body, produces fresh blood, cleanses the body, produces glowing skin, and provides nutrients for healthy eyes and liver. For those that have health issues, carrot juice daily is a must to help bring the body back to health.

Its juice helps you maintain the proper balance between alkaline and acid body. Because of its high vitamin A and E, carrot juice is effective in promoting bones and teeth and most importantly the maintenance of healthy body tissues and glandular function. It also has vitamin B, C, D, and K. Pregnant women should include carrot juice in their diet and during nursing for their health and for the health of the baby.

You can take carrot juice indefinitely and in any reasonable quantity – 1 to 4 pints a day is ok. If you have digestion or appetite problems, carrot juice is a must. If you need help in keeping your teeth healthy, carrot juice will help improve your jaw and teeth structure.

Celery Juice

This has a high level of potassium. If you need potassium, then this is the juice to drink. You can add carrot juice to this juice to make it more palatable. Celery juice is also high in sodium and is considered an alkaline food.

If you frequently feel nervous or agitated, try drinking a combination of celery and carrot juice. This combination is good for restoring the function of degenerating nerve sheathing.

Ginger

Ginger can give you temporary relief for acid reflux. Mix 1/2 tsp. of powdered ginger or 1 1/2 tsp. of fresh ginger in 8 oz. of boiling water. Add a bit of honey to make it more drinkable.

Chamomile

Chamomile has been used frequently for heartburn and hiatus hernia. It provides a soothing effect on your stomach and overall body. Prepare it in the following way:

- Boil water and place it into a cup
- Add one teaspoon of chamomile flowers or use a tea bag.
- Let tea sit for 5 minutes
- Add a little honey for better taste
- Drink tea when still warm.
- Drink tea 3 times a day and between meals.

Cinnamon

Cinnamon is a natural remedy that has been used for soothing the stomach. It can relieve stomach pain and bloating. It also has antacid properties. Here is how to use it.

- Add 1/2 teaspoon of powdered cinnamon to a cup hot water.

- Let the tea sit for 5 minutes.

- Drink your tea while it is warm and 2-3 times a day.

Warm Water Remedy

First thing in the morning drink a glass of warm water. Then follow this up with an exercise that is outlined in chapter 11.

This chapter has a lot of juices you can make. Choose one or two and start drinking them. Then choose new fruits in the weeks that come.

11: Supplements That Help Eliminate Hiatus Hernia

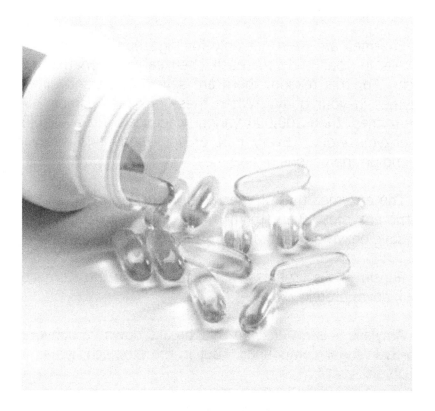

Enzymes

When you have hiatus hernia, you want to have the best digestion possible. You need to be taking digestive enzymes. Enzymes are proteins that accelerate food digestion. They bring food molecules close together and create an environment that results in the intended reaction. They basically lower the energy required for a chemical reaction to take place – activation energy.

Enzymes can also digest the stomach lining, if the lining is not protected as in the existence of a stomach ulcer. For this reason, enzymes are released as needed by nerve and hormonal activities.

Enzymes are used not only for digestion but are used in all cells in your body for each chemical reaction that takes place. For this reason, there are several thousand different enzymes in your body. When these enzymes combine with co-enzymes, then 100,000 various chemicals are available to do enzyme work. Every part of your body and every cell depend on the actions of enzymes.

The enzymes that are secreted in the stomach are called gastric enzymes. The stomach contains the following gastric digestive enzymes, acid, and substances:

Pepsin – is a protease that is released in the stomach to break down protein.

Amylase – is an enzyme that breaks down carbohydrates into their sugar compounds. But in the stomach, it has little activity.

Gelatinase – breaks down certain types of gelatin and collagen found in meat

Lipase – is call tributyrase and is an enzyme that works exclusively on tributyrin, a fat found in butter that is used in the production of margarine.

It also contains HCl and intrinsic factor.

Taking enzyme supplements

It is important to be taking **digestive enzymes** with each meal. Digestive enzymes can be taken by young children, but are especially needed by all adults.

The reason you should take digestive enzymes at any age is that most food that you eat is cooked and this destroys the food's natural digestive enzymes. This puts a load on your body to create and bring into the various digestive area enzymes to digest the food you have eaten.

Loss of enzyme power

Every ten years of your life you lose 13% of your power to create enzymes. So at the age of 60, you have lost around 50 - 60% of your ability to produce enzymes. By this time, most people are exhibiting illnesses that relate to lack of specific minerals, vitamins or nutrients. Up to 50% of all adults do not produce enough digestive enzymes to digest all the food they eat.

There are two types of enzymes – digestive and systemic. The digestive enzymes are used to digest your food. You can get digestive enzymes by eating raw food – fruits and vegetables. When you eat processed food, your body has to supply the enzymes. When your body is deficient in digestive enzymes, your body has to use systemic enzymes that are used for various body chemical reactions to keep your body healthy.

Digestive Enzymes to Use

Look for digestive enzymes that have pepsin, amylase, and lipase. You may also want to try some digestive enzymes that contain betaine HCl, hydrochloric acid. Adding more acid,

HCl, to your stomach may be important if you have been using OTC drugs or if your natural production of HCl has decreased.

To make your enzymes more effective, chew your food completely. If you are in a hurry during your meals, you will not be chewing your food for the right time. When you do not break down your food in your mouth, whole pieces of food will enter your stomach.

Stomach and small intestine enzymes will only be able to dissolve the outer the area of that food, causing undigested food to enter your colon. This undigested food is the source for bad colon bacterial to multiple. When bad bacteria dominate your colon, you open yourself to poor health.

Probiotic

By taking a probiotic you can improve your digestion. Start by using a probiotic that contains 4 billion active organisms. Look for a brand that contains lactobacillus, acidophilus and bifidus. Using unsweetened yogurt or kefir is recommended.

Papaya Enzymes

Use papaya enzymes or fresh papaya for increasing your digestive power. Papaya helps you to digest more protein, which helps you improve your cell regeneration abilities. You need strong cells and tissue to help you get rid of Hiatus Hernia.

Use to 2 to 3 papaya tablets before meals or eat some papaya fruit before or after your meal.

If you like papaya and have it available, eat fresh papaya.

You can add it to your morning fruit breakfast or to your fruit smoothies.

Licorice Root (DGL)

Take licorice root in the form of DGL. This herbal product comes in chewable tables. Take one tablet 20 minutes before meals. This herb will soothe and heal the stomach and esophagus. Take only three times a week and only for one month. Use daily as instructed on the bottle. This is an important herb to take.

Use of DGL is helpful in eliminating or controlling the H. Pylori bacteria. H. Pylori affect the health of your stomach and cause acid reflux.

Orange Peels

Orange peels seasoning has helped many people with mild and severe acid reflux and hiatus hernia. In some cases, it has interfered with sleep. Orange peel can be bought in most health food stores or on the internet in 16 oz. bottles. You can sprinkle it on your morning fruit, cereal, or toast. Use it where you can accept the taste, and for at least twice a day.

Slippery Elm or Marshmallow Root

Both of these herbs will help reduce the inflammation of your stomach and esophagus lining. Take 300mg two to three times a day of each herb. Reducing inflammation helps power up your immune system.

Slippery elm can also be used as a tea. It has been found good for reducing heartburn and stomach acid. It is known for providing anti-inflammatory properties for digestive problems.

In a cup of hot water add one tablespoon of slippery elm bark powder and let it sit for 10 minutes. Drink twice a day after meals.

Vitamin A Emulsion

Use 50,000 IU for the first month, then drop down to 30,000 IU for two weeks. Use 20,000 IU after that.

Using vitamin A emulsion is better than using the pill form since it gets into your body quicker to the healing process.

Vitamin B

Take two capsules of multivitamin Vitamin B 100 each day, once in the morning and in the evening with meals. If you have been using various OTC drugs that lower your stomach acid, you can take a sublingual B12 vitamin to bypass your stomach. Also, you can take one B12 lozenge during the day. You can't overdose on B12, since the excess turns your urine yellow, showing the excess is being eliminated.

Adding some addition niacinamide, Vitamin B3, in addition to the B100 multivitamins, has been found to be useful for hiatus. Use around 700mg per day of B3.

Potassium

When using potassium supplements always take them with meals. Potassium requires other minerals and vitamins to be present for adequate digestion and adsorption. The actual form you use is important so that your body will be able to absorb it.

Here are three types of potassium you can buy.

Potassium glycerophosphate – is one of the best forms of potassium, since it is easily and quickly absorbed by your body and cell walls.

Potassium citrate – is readily absorbed, and it is useful in restoring urinary citrate back to normal. Citrate is important because it reduces the formation of calcium salt stones. In the urine, citrate can be reduced when you eat excess sodium and protein. In addition, Potassium citrate reduces urinary calcium excretion, which helps lessen the loss of calcium.

Potassium aspartate – is a form where potassium is tied to the aspartic acid, which is an acidic amino acid. When minerals are tied to amino acids, they pass easily and quickly through your intestinal wall and into your bloodstream.

When taking potassium supplements, make sure the formulation also has magnesium. Magnesium is necessary to maintain potassium in the body. Also, your heart muscle will not hold potassium without the presence of magnesium.

Vitamin C

Take 500 mg of buffered vitamin C every day. Always include vitamin C in your daily supplements. Your body is always in need of vitamin C.

Zinc

Zinc is an important mineral to take and is necessary for any healing and repair of tissue that has been damaged by your hiatus hernia.

Use only 50 mg per day.

Magnesium

Use about 1000:500 mg of calcium-magnesium to help tighten the esophagus and stomach muscles.

Apple Cider Vinegar

Apple cider vinegar can be helpful in getting quick relief from acid reflux and hiatus hernia issues. If you have been taking drugs that lower your stomach acid, then apple cider vinegar will bring back some of your stomach acids. You can test, using 1 to 1 ½ tablespoon of cider in 8 oz. of lukewarm water, to see if cider will be effective. Take small sips of this mixture just before meals.

Homeopathic Nux Vomica

Using homeopathic medicine in conjunction to all other remedies here can help you get your body back into balance. Nux Vomica is used for acid reflux and heartburn, which occurs from stress, spicy foods, and alcohol. Use a 30C potency two to three times a day. You will find homeopathic remedies at many health food stores. Or go to a homeopathic doctor to get other homeopathic medication to help with your other hiatus hernia symptoms.

Additional good food to eat:
- Cucumbers, asparagus, leafy greens

- Berries, melons

- Parsley, fennel, ginger

- Bone Broth

- Yogurt

- Aloe Vera

Aloe vera has anti-bacterial, anti-inflammatory, and cell regeneration properties. This is an excellent herb to add to your approach to hiatus hernia. By drinking this herb, you can coat any esophagus tissue damage you might have from acid reflux. In addition, taking a capsule, you can get stomach relief and decrease any constipation issues you might have.

You can buy ready-made aloe vera drink, or you can make it yourself as follows:

- Extract gel from a fresh Aloe Vera leaf or purchase gel that is 98 to 99 %.
- Blend two tablespoons or less
- Add 8 oz. of fresh orange juice to aloe in the blender
- Drink 1/4 cup of this blend, 20 minutes before eating your lunch or dinner.

12: Why Vitamin D3 is Necessary for Hiatus Hernia

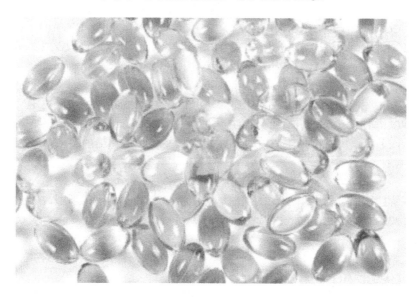

Vitamin D3, the Hormone

The use of vitamin D3 therapy is critical in any nutritional program. It brings in more calcium, magnesium, and other minerals into your body to strengthen your body muscles, tissues, and bones. Because you will absorb more calcium when you take vitamin D3, you will need vitamin K2 to route the calcium to the places where your body needs it.

D3 with calcium and magnesium are involved in thousands of chemical reactions in your body. With more calcium and magnesium going where it should in your body, you improve your chances of eliminating your acid body and creating an alkaline body.

Vitamin D3 is considered a hormone and not a vitamin. It was mislabel a vitamin, during the time it was discovered, since it was thought to come from food. The vitamin form that is active in your body is Vitamin D3, known as cholecalciferol. Vitamin D3 is tasked with communicating with your DNA. It turns on and off over 1000 genes to activate their function.

There is also vitamin D2, which is considerably less active in your body. D3 is around 300% more active in your body than D2. Most foods that are fortified with vitamin D use the D2 form.

Vitamin D3 is created when UV light activates a conversion form of cholesterol, which occurs in or on your skin.

D3 Helps Absorb Calcium

Another vitamin D3 function is to help you absorb calcium. Calcium aside from helping to form bone structures is a key mineral in helping to keep your body alkaline. An alkaline body is the natural state of your body, and an acid body is a state of disease. You can gain more information on how to maintain an alkaline body in my ebook called "**Alkaline Body**"

How Much Vitamin D3 do You Need?

So, what is the dose for vitamin D3? During the 30's and 40's studies showed that taking more than 50,000 IU was still safe. However, pharmaceuticals went on a scare tactic by saying that taking more than 400 IU of vitamin D was toxic.

Yet, being out in the sun for 30 minutes can produce 10,000 to 20,000 IU of vitamin D3.

When vitamin D3 was demonized during the 40's, the pharmaceuticals came out with three miracle drugs for treating various deadly diseases. These drugs were nothing more than 50,000 IU of vitamin D.

The amount of vitamin D3 you may need will depend on a couple of factors. The more obese you are the more D3 you need. You can experiment on how much you need by seeing what result you get with different doses. Take a certain amount for 3 to 4 weeks to see if your health improves.

You can start as follows:

- Normal weight – 5,000 to 10,000 IU

- Overweight – 8,000 to 12,000

- Obese – 8,000 to 15,000

If you take over 10,000 IU of vitamin D3, you will have to supplement with vitamin 1000 mcg of K2 to avoid calcium depositing in body tissue and joints.

You should be ok to take up to and more than 20,000 IU of vitamin D3. To do this you must take a minimum of 1000 mcg of vitamin K2 per 10,000 IU of vitamin D3. Be sure not to take too much K2, since it can cause a racing heart or high blood pressure. If this happens, you would then just back off on the K2, until those symptoms disappear.

Doses of 8,000 IU, in studies, did not exhibit excess calcium in the blood. The additional calcium brought into the blood by high D3 supplementation was found to be properly used by the body.

Because D3 is fat soluble, you can optimize its adsorption by taking a healthy fat with it.

Calcium, Vitamin D3, and K2

Vitamin D3 helps to move calcium passed your small intestinal barrier and into your blood. Vitamin K2 then moves the calcium to the right areas of your body. K2 prevents calcium from building up along your arteries and accumulating in your soft tissue and bones.

Types of Vitamin K

There are several kinds of vitamin K. There are K1 and K2, where K2 has several forms of which K7 is the most active and important form. K2 (MK-4) is usually used in high doses of 1000mcg per 10,000 D3 doses. However, K7 is used in smaller doses of 100 to 200 mcg per 10,000mg of D3.

Aside from vitamin D3 being necessary for proper calcium absorption, strong bones, teeth, immune system, heart health, it is also useful in the prevention of cancer and other diseases. Low levels of Vitamin D3 are associated with almost every disease you develop.

In the NaturalHealth365 website article, Lori Alton, staff writer, writes,

"According to the Institute of Medicine, 4,000 IU daily is the tolerable upper level of intake – defined as the highest level that would be unlikely to cause harm to nearly all adults. However, the Vitamin D Council recommends that adults take 5,000 IU of the vitamin a day.

Meanwhile, a naturopathic practitioner might advise dosages in the area of 8,000 IU of vitamin D a day, depending on the individual's history and lifestyle. The Endocrine Society Practice Guidelines maintain that adults can safely take up to 10,000 IU a day – more than double what the IOM advises as the safe upper level.

Bottom line: ensuring that you have adequate levels of vitamin D3 just might be one of the most important things you can do to protect your health – and your life."

The supplement to take is one that has calcium, magnesium, vitamin D3, and vitamin K. If you can't find such a supplement, build one from single nutrients. To enhance the effectiveness of vitamin D3, take fish or coconut oil pill.

Simply by increasing your blood levels of D3, you give yourself protection against various diseases. Optimum blood levels of D3 are **50 ng/ml to 80 ng/ml**

Respiratory Infections

In a study made at Queen Mary University in London, researchers found that Vitamin D3 was just as effective as getting a flu shot in protecting against a respiratory infection. It was found that Vitamin D3 produces over 210 antimicrobials.

Immune System

It has been discovered that Vitamin D receptors have been found in all immune cells. Further studies show that various autoimmune disorders benefit from increased Vitamin D3 supplementation.

Heart Disease

Low levels of blood vitamin D3 have been associated with cardiovascular and stroke issues. Higher levels of D3 are related to the lowest risks of heart attack, stroke, and death.

Magnesium

Magnesium is necessary for calcium to function properly in your body. It also activates enzymes that help your body use vitamin D3. Without magnesium, vitamin D3 cannot be used by your body. For this reason, it is not a good idea to take calcium without magnesium, vitamin D3, and vitamin K2.

To get many of the other minerals that aid in the proper function of calcium, D3, and K2, eat those foods that are high in magnesium.

Nutrients Needed by Vitamin D3

There are many other nutrients that interact with D3. These can come from your diet. Vitamin A, zinc, and boron are few important ones.

Food That Has D3

Very little D3 is found in food. The foods that have some D3 are eggs, wild cold water fish, and organic mushrooms, soy (non GMO), unsweetened yogurt, and ricotta cheese.

Final Words on Vitamin D3

Many studies have been done on vitamin D3 and have substantiated the need to use it in doses up to 10,000 IU or more. The recommended RDA of 400 IU is totally out of line with the body's need for this vitamin, especially if you are sick.

In combination with calcium, magnesium, and K2, vitamin D3 emerges as the nutrient required in large quantities necessary for quality health.

Studies have shown that healthy blood levels of Vitamin D3 are in the range of 50 to 80 ng/ml. Blood level below 30 ng/ml has always shown to be associated with all kinds of disease. The amount of vitamin D3 required for good health has been established to be 5,000 to 10,000 IU of vitamin D3.

Here is the recommended supplement program by Robert R. Barefoot, Nutritionist and BioChemist, as stated in his 2002 book, Death by Diet.

The pH listed below is based on your saliva test listed in this book.

pH	calcium	magnesium	vit. D3	vit. A
6.5 to 7.4	1200mg	690mg	2400IU	30000IU
6.0 to 6.5	2400mg	1380mg	4800IU	60000IU
4.5 TO 6.0	3600mg	2070mg	7200IU	90000IU

The pH listed in the above chart is associated with the following body conditions.

- pH 6.5 to 7.4 is the normal body condition

- pH 6.0 to 6.5 is where the body is developing a disease

- pH 4.5 to 6.0 is where you have a disease

Vitamin K

If you take less than 10,000 mg of vitamin D3, you may not need to take any vitamin K. But, if you are taking 10,000 IU or more, you should take 1000mcg of K2 with some 100mcg of k7. The k7 is much stronger than the K1 or K2.

Side effects of Vitamin K

Some people have to experience Vitamin K side effects when they have taken too much. These side effects are high blood pressure, headaches, racing heart, and so on. When you experience these side effects, simply back off on the amount of vitamin K you are taking, until the side effect disappear.

13: Exercises Needed To Eliminate Hiatus Hernia

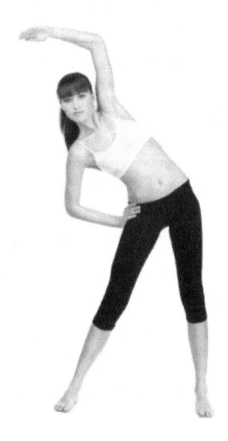

Chiropractic adjustment

This is not an exercise, but a movement of muscles, tissues, and vertebras along your spine.

In her book, Digestive Wellness by Elizabeth Lipski, M.S.C.C.N., 1996, says,

"Seek chiropractic care for hiatal hernia. Cranial-sacral adjustments can often correct gastric reflux, especially in children. Chiropractic or osteopathic adjustment is often all the therapy you need for these problems."

In their book called, Prescription for Natural Cures, James F. Balch, M.D. and Mark Stengler, N.D., 2004, recommends,

"A chiropractor, an osteopath, or a naturopath can perform a gentle manipulation of your stomach with a downward pull. This helps reduce the stomach protrusion and soft tissues that have gone too far up through the diaphragm. Noticeable improvements can be noted within a few treatments.

Also, acupuncture can be quite effective in managing the symptoms."

A true cure comes from diet correction and changes in the way you live. A chiropractic adjustment can give you a new start if your hernia is not severe. Chiropractic adjustments are always a powerful way to correct health issues.

To perform a simple abdominal self-massage, follow the steps below:

- Look for a flat surface to lie on. This could be your bed or on the floor.

- Assume a supine position by lying on your back. Try to be as relaxed as possible.

- Locate your sternum or your breastbones and put your finger below this area.

- Apply a moderate pressure and slowly move your fingers towards your navel or belly button. Remember to maintain moderate pressure as you slide your fingers down.

- Do this for 5 whole minutes.

- Perform the abdominal self-massage two times a day, preferably in the morning and in the evening.

Yoga

For Hiatus Hernia you will need to do exercises that tone your abdomen area. And, you cannot just do 10 minutes of exercise. You need to do at least 10 to 30 minutes of exercise. This will help to tone up your abdominal muscles and other parts of the body. The exercise that is best for toning the whole body is yoga. However, if you have not done yoga before, then start slowly, with a few movements and work up to longer sessions. Only do the following yoga moves and avoid the others.

- Raised legs pose
- Wind-relieving pose
- Chair Pose

These poses will help you strengthen your stomach and LES valve.

Lying Exercise

Look into a yoga book and do those exercises that are done with you lying on your back and where you need to move in certain ways to strengthen your abdominal muscles – sit-up type movements. Also look for exercises with other positions that will help you exercise your abdomen.

Lying on your back, you can raise both legs up to a 45-degree angle or even to a 90 degree, and then move your legs down to the floor. Do 10 of these movements in the beginning and gradually increase the number.

Lying on your back, you raise your legs to 90 degrees. Then move them constantly by Criss-Crossing them from left to right. Move your right leg to the left and the left leg to the right at the same time. You will be able to feel the tension in your abdominal area. Start with a few of these and gradually work up.

The Criss Cross, exercise helps to build your abs. It works on the oblique abdominal muscles that help stabilize your posture and aid in forward bending and rotation of the spine.

Sitting Exercise

Sitting on a chair twist your body left as you look over your shoulder. Then move your body to the right as you look over your shoulder again. Do this at least 10 times when you first start.

Sitting on a chair, bend forward with arms stretched out to touch the floor. Sit up and then bend forward again. These exercises, again, work your abdomen.

Sitting on a chair, place your hands behind your neck. Pull your head forward towards your stomach and hold for a few seconds. Then, move your head and hands back to their original position. Repeat for 10 times.

Here is a breathing exercise recommended by Richard Firshein, D.O., assistant professor of family medicine at the New York College of Osteopathic Medicine in New York,

"Lie on your back and place a book on your abdomen. As you inhale and exhale, the book should move up and down several inches. Continue this deep-breathing exercise for several minutes or until you feel some relief. This exercise helps to strengthen the diaphragm and reinforce the hiatal opening."

Wait about two hours after eating to do this exercise.

Walking

However, walking briskly is also a great exercise. It is best to start with a short walk of about 10 minutes and gradually work up your time each day. Walk fast enough to create a sweat. Don't start off with a long walk where you get tired and don't want to walk again the next day.

Sweating helps you get rid of toxins. This is part of your program to eliminate toxins from your body. When you do this, your cells and tissue work better and become normal. Toxins are part of what made your LES and stomach lining weak.

All that you have read here is to assist your body in getting rid of toxins. Your body is always working toward the elimination of toxins and waste material through the elimination of urine, feces, and sweat. By having good nutrition from a good diet, using the body cycles, and spending time exercising, you can help your body recover from Hiatus Hernia.

Rebounding or Heel Exercise

Here is a great exercise to do that will help you to manage or get rid of your hiatus hernia. It has a lot of benefits for getting you healthy again.

Drink 8 to 16 oz. of **warm water** when you first wake up. Get on a rebounder or trampoline, if you have one, and rebound for about 10 minutes. At first, you might start with 5 minutes. This will help you pull your stomach down and strengthen all of your muscles around your abdomen.

Without the rebounder, you can do the following. After drinking your water, here's what to do:

In a standing position, stretch your arm straight out in front of you. Now bend your arm so your hands come together at your chest. The will open your hiatus and stretch your diaphragm

Now, rise on your toes, then, drop fast to your heels. Do this 5 to 10 times. As days pass add a few more cycles. When you do this, you will pull down on your water filled stomach. It's best to use tongs and not shoes.

To end the routine, stand straight with arms straight up and breathe with short and rapid cycles, with your mouth open. Do this for 15 seconds.

There you have it, exercises to do. Vary the exercises you do, so that you can stretch and exercise different muscles and tissues related to your abdominal area

14: About The Hiatus Hernia Author

Rudy Silva is a natural nutritional consultant educated in the United States in Nutrition and Physics. He is a graduate of San Jose State University in California. He is the author of 40 other books on natural remedies. He has authored a newsletter in natural remedies for over 10 years.

Resource page

Check the internet for his other kindle books on natural remediesr.

If you need support or want to promote any of his books, please contact him at rss41@yahoo.com.

Give A Review

And, don't forget to give a review for this book. It's not hard to give a review. It can be only a sentence or two. You don't have to leave a long review. A short review helps other people decide if they want to buy a book. So give a short review and give your thoughts to help other people and to help the author improve his book.

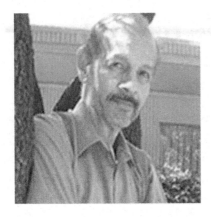

To you, for creating better health and more happiness,

Rudy S Silva

Made in United States
Orlando, FL
11 November 2021